D1408618

36½ Reasons to Laugh

Published exclusively for Johnson & Johnson Healthcare Products Division of McNEIL-PPC, Inc., by Chronicle Books LLC.

Text copyright © McNEIL-PPC, Inc. 2009
Illustrations © 2009 by Chuck Gonzales/artcounselinc.com

All rights reserved. No part of this book may be reproduced in any form without written permission from the publisher.

ISBN: 978-0-8118-7278-2

Library of Congress Cataloging-in-Publication Data available.

Manufactured in the United States of America.

Design by Elizabeth Van Itallie.
This book has been set in Futura.
Photograph on page 7 by Blake Little.

LISTERINE® and REACH® are registered trademarks of Johnson & Johnson.

Use LISTERINE® and REACH® products as directed.

*While the National Children's Oral Health Foundation®: America's Toothfairy is referenced in this book,
the organization's inclusion is not an endorsement of any of the products or content in the book.*

10 9 8 7 6 5 4 3 2 1

Chronicle Books LLC
680 Second Street
San Francisco, CA 94107

www.chroniclebooks.com

36½ Reasons to Laugh

A SLICE OF LIFE

WRITTEN BY RICK ADAMS
ILLUSTRATED BY CHUCK GONZALES
FOREWORD BY DOUG SAVANT

CHRONICLE BOOKS
SAN FRANCISCO

CONTENTS

FOREWORD

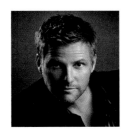

In all my years as an actor and a dad, I've learned that laughter really is the great connector. When I'm on set, joking around brings the cast and crew together and makes those twelve-hour shoots more bearable. At home with my four kids, I can always count on someone to say or do something funny (usually unintentionally), and we share a lot of laughs.

The funniest moments always seem to come from the most mundane situations. That's what this book is all about: the hilarious ups and downs that life throws at us every day. I think you'll recognize a lot of these moments, and you'll nod a lot while you're laughing.

I love the Family chapter of this book—it reminds me of my own brood. "The Family Plan" on page 11 really hits home. Like any family, mine is learning how to balance quality time with technology time—guess which is still winning? I also feel for the guy on page 65—that's the only way my wife could get me to go to yoga, too!

Not only will this book bring a smile to your face, it's also literally giving new smiles to kids across America. In support of this book, the makers of LISTERINE® TOTAL CARE are helping the National Children's Oral Health Foundation®: America's Toothfairy provide dental care to kids in need. Having a healthy smile is every child's right—and that's no joke.

Now turn the page and start laughing!

Doug Savant

FAMILY

The Family Plan

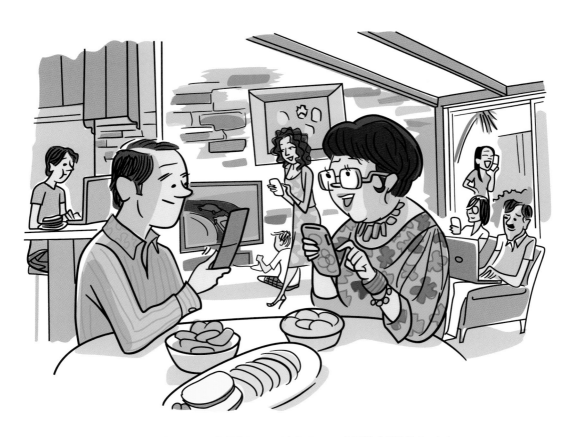

I . . . LUV . . . THESE . . . FMLY . . . GET2GETHRS :-) !

Old School vs. New Skool

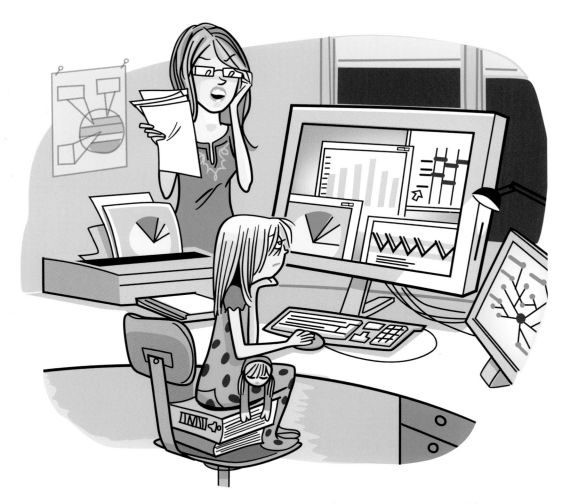

"No, Britney! You CAN'T go to bed until you finish Mommy's spreadsheet!"

Our Dad's Electric!

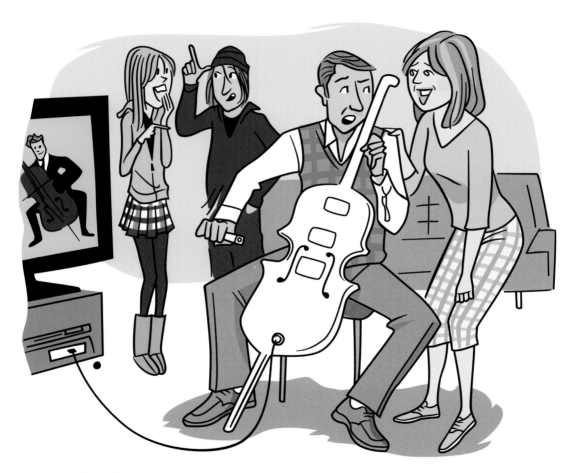

"I don't think you're really selling them on the 'Cello Hero' game, dear . . ."

Brace Yourself

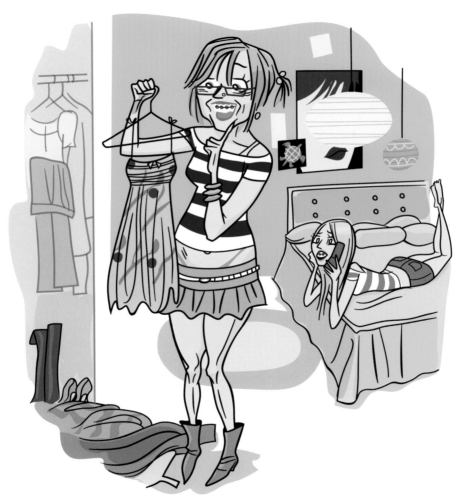

"Ever since my mom and I got matching braces, she thinks she can raid my closet!"

Bill Board

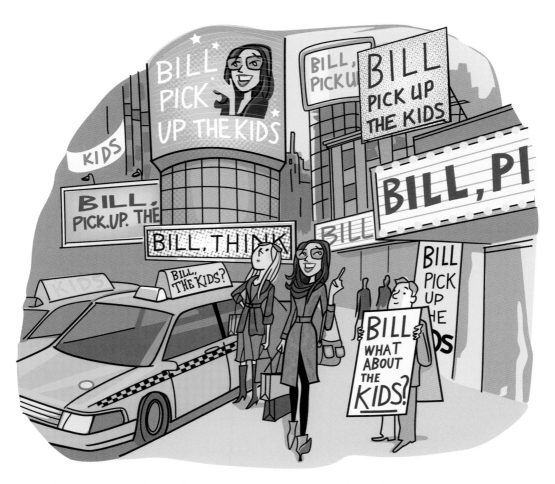

"It's expensive, but at least he never forgets to pick up the kids from school!"

How Kids *Really* See Their Parents

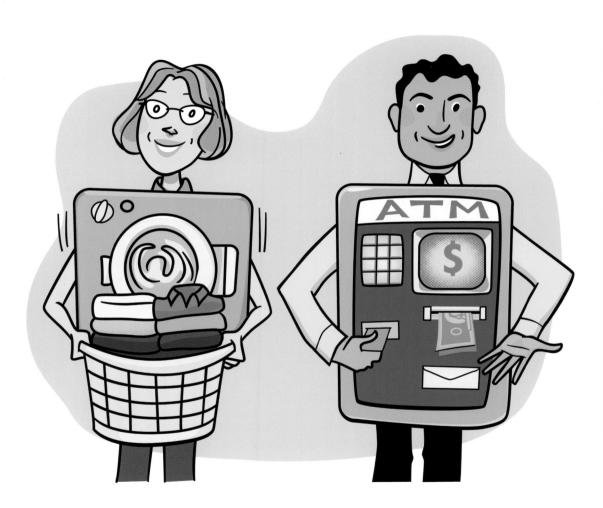

Operation Diaper Change

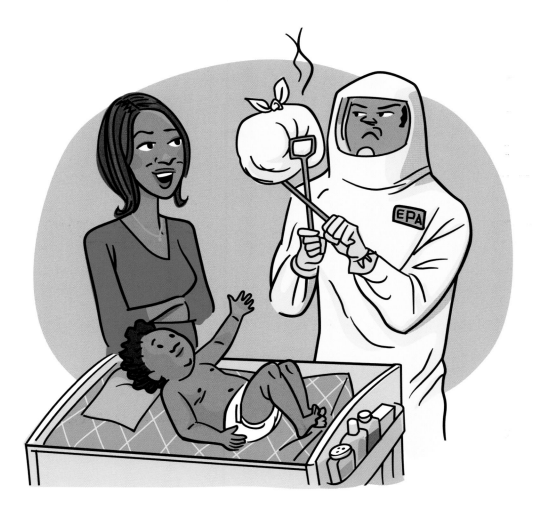

"Honestly, Ainsley! I know you work for the E.P.A., but don't you think you're taking your turn to change the diaper a little TOO seriously?"

Recognizing Your Teenager's Moods

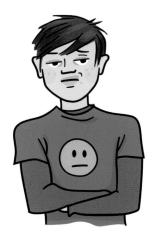

HAPPY

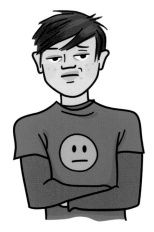

SAD

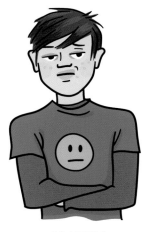

ANGRY

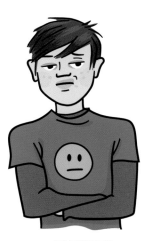

EXCITED

Get the Massage?

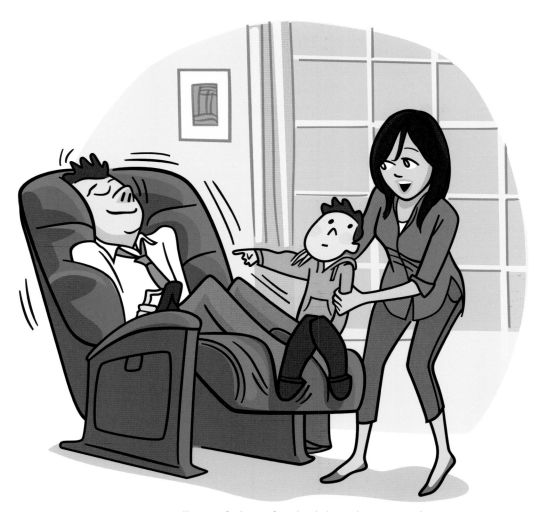

"No, Ryan! Wait till your father's finished the 'I hate my job' setting."

OFFICE

Ease of Communication

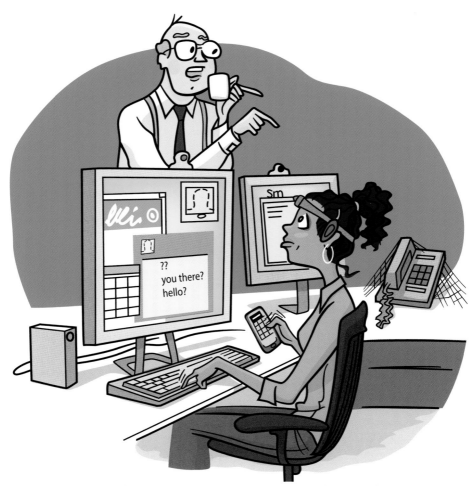

"So you tried instant messaging, texting, emailing, and posting on his blog . . . but did you try calling him?"

I ♥ My Manager!

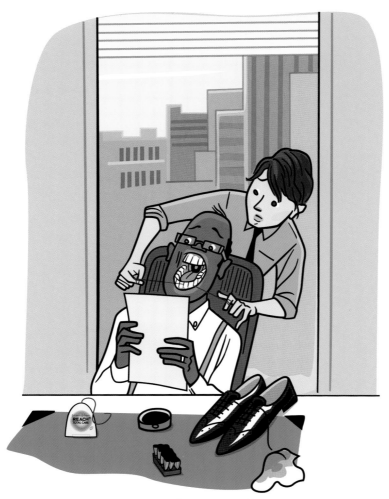

"Nice sucking up, Jackson!"

Free Food!

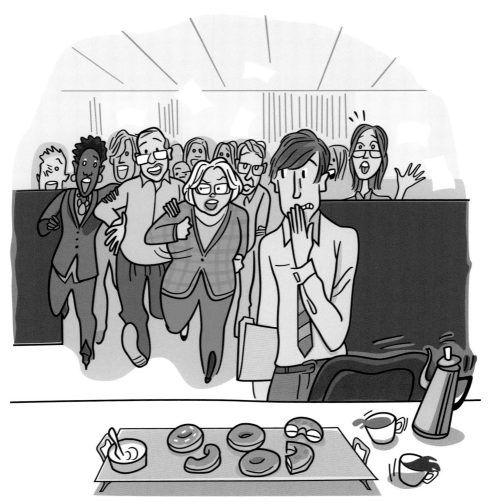

Next time Malcolm will say "free bagels" a little more quietly . . .

Carpool

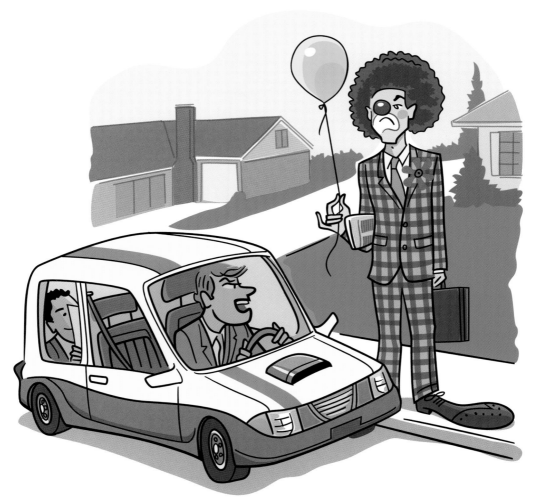

"Yeah, yeah! So it's a SMALL car—you've made your point—GET IN!"

The Joy of Email

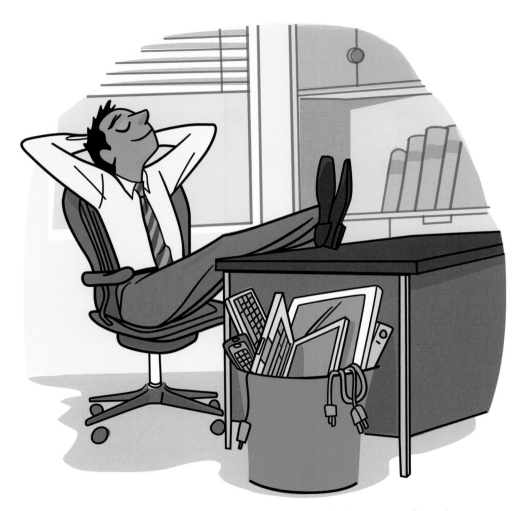

Robert finally found the perfect way to deal with the spam in his inbox.

Office Ergonomics

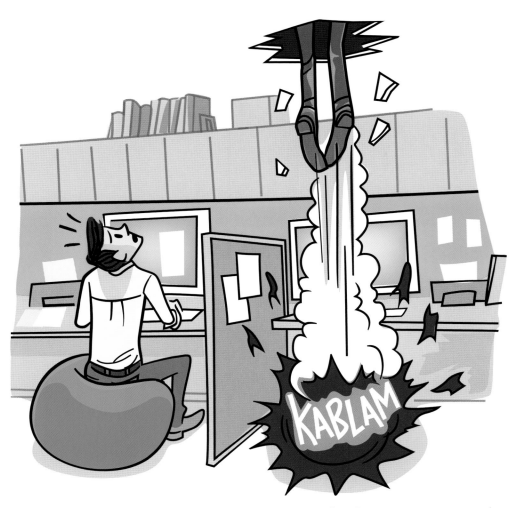

"I hate these fancy new office seats . . . but at least they keep your spine straight!"

ENTERTAI

NMENT

Death by Popcorn

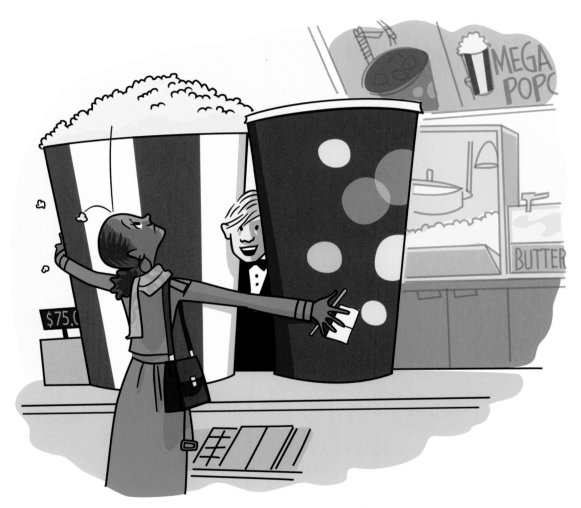

"Would you like to supersize your order, ma'am?"

How Mini Golf *Really* Works

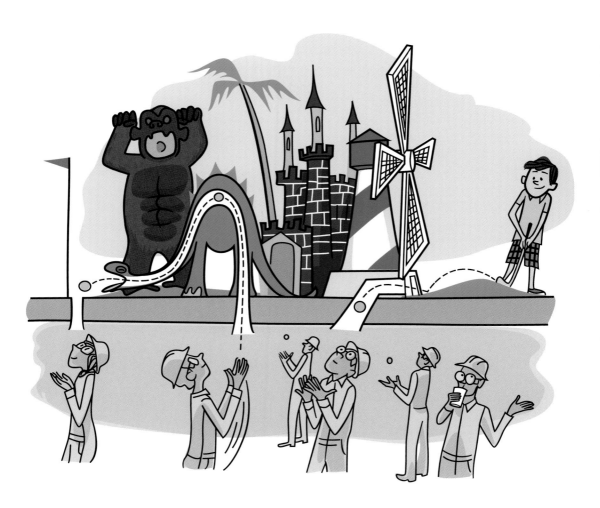

Extreme Sports

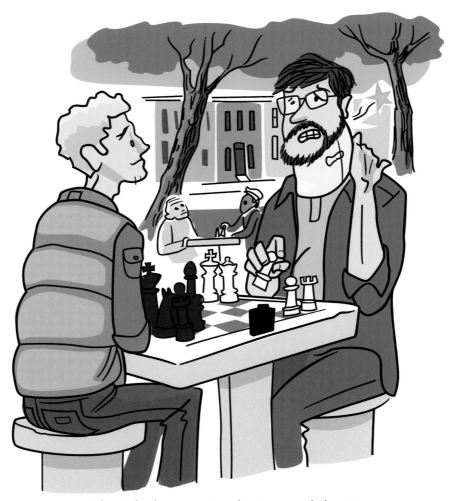

"That's the last time I'm playing speed chess!"

Renaissance Fair

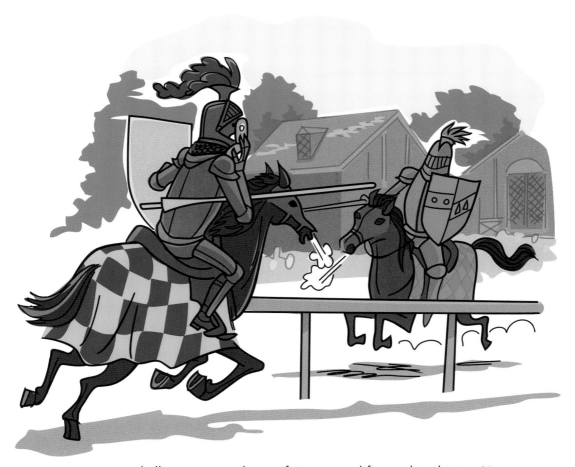

"Yes . . . hello, I was wondering if I'm covered for medieval injury?"

HEALTHY LIVING

The Chiropractor

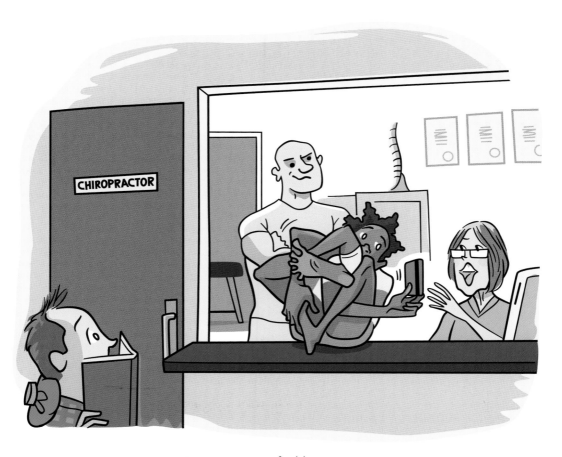

"See? Don't you feel better now?"

Downward Ugh!

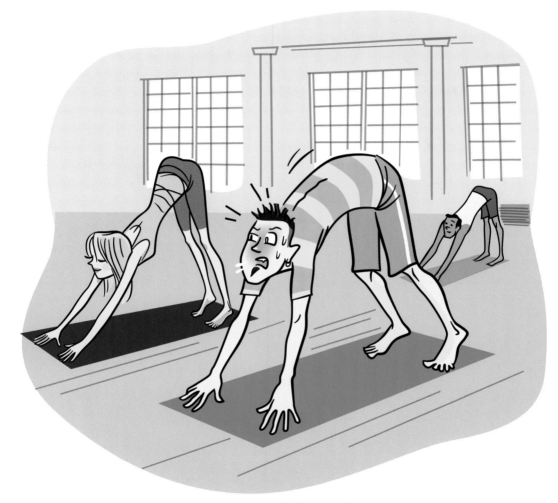

Micah's Downward Dog looked more like Dyspeptic Cat!

My Mom's a Health Nut!

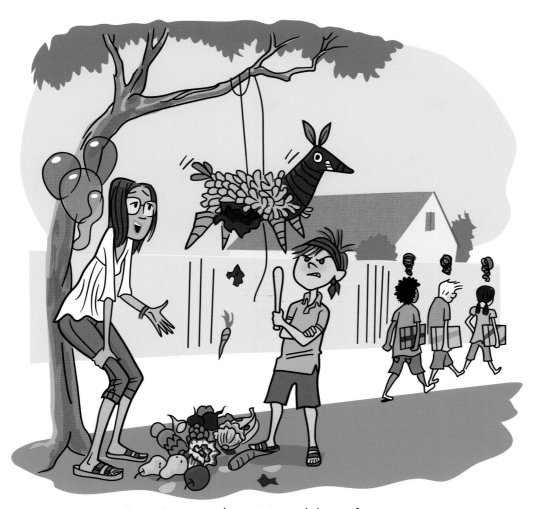

"But, Georgie—this is SO much better for you!"

Bio Phewwwel

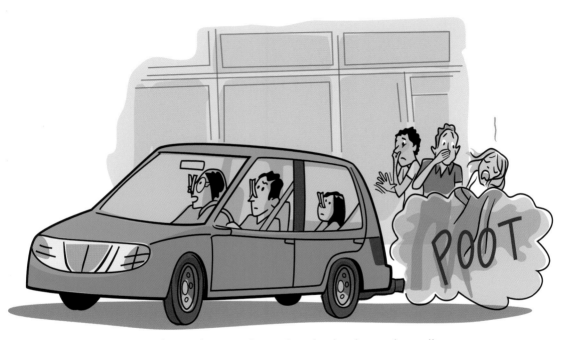

Forty miles an hour with two hundred miles to the gallon!
Everything was looking good for Todd's brussels-sprout-and-broccoli-powered car!

Overbite

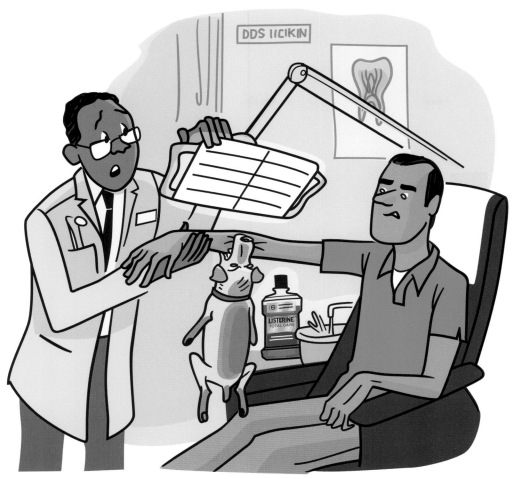

"When you said you had canine teeth that needed removing,
this wasn't quite what I had in mind!"

Namas . . . Hey!

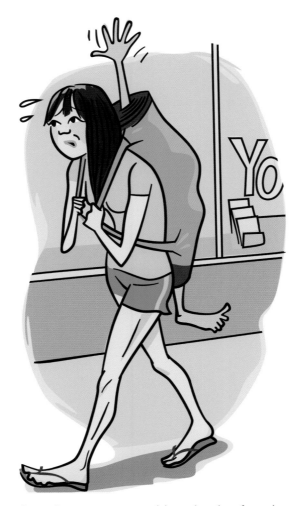

Sadly, this was the only way Mary could get her boyfriend to go to yoga.

Personal Strainer

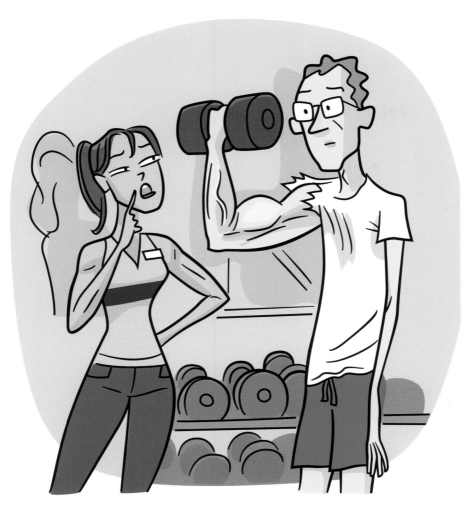

"OK, I think we can move to the other arm now."

RELATION

SHIPS

Online Dating

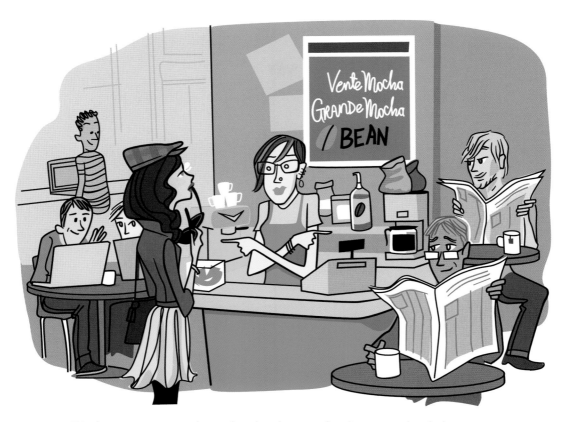

"E_dating.com over there, lovehookup.net by the stairs, hunkylove.com by the window . . . or have you just come for coffee?"

Like Cats and Dogs

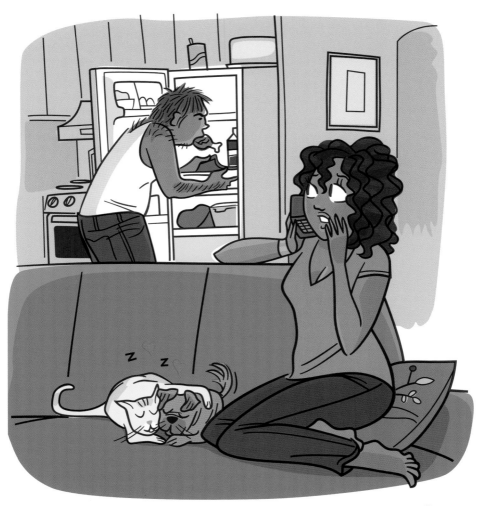

"I'd dump him in a heartbeat, Anne, but our pets get along SO well!"

I Love You—What?!

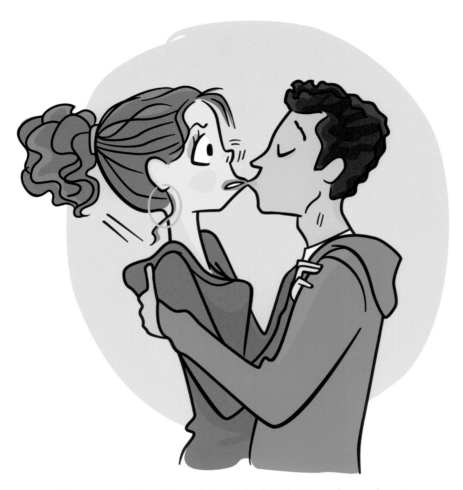

Bergamot with a hint of lime? Suddenly Tracy knew that Roger
was getting his mouthwash from someone else!

Bedtime Performance Art

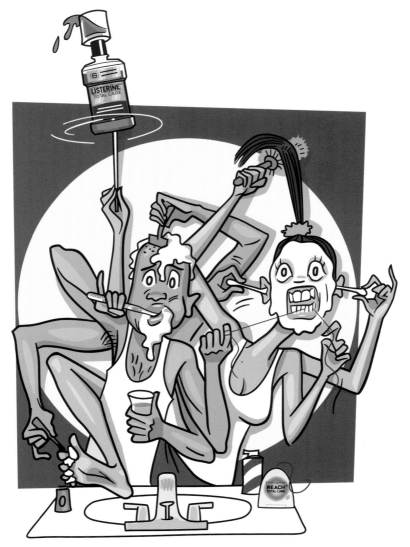

Eye Like You

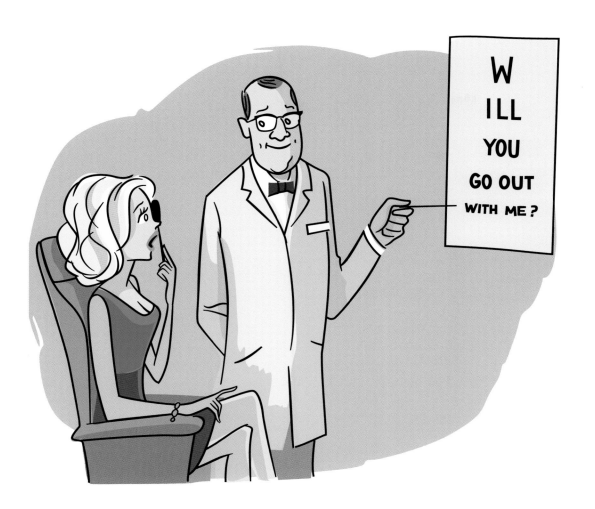

ETCETERA

The Magic Show

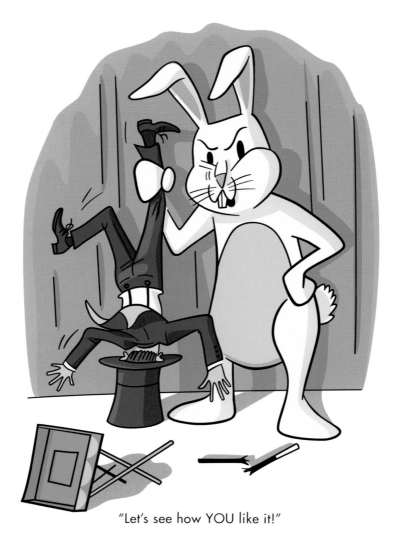

"Let's see how YOU like it!"

Road to Nowhere

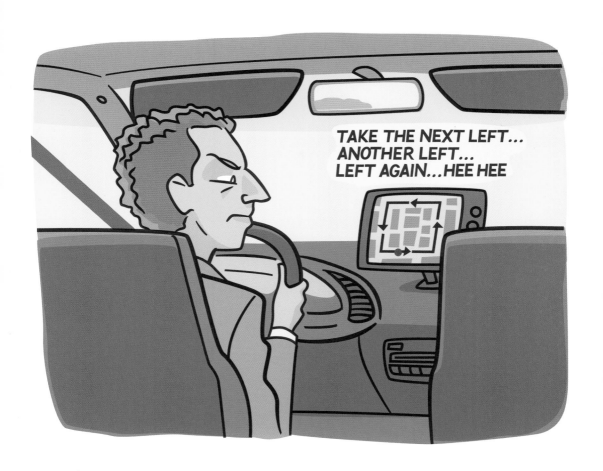

If Geoff didn't know better, he would have the distinct impression
that his GPS was messing with him.

How Sushi Was Invented

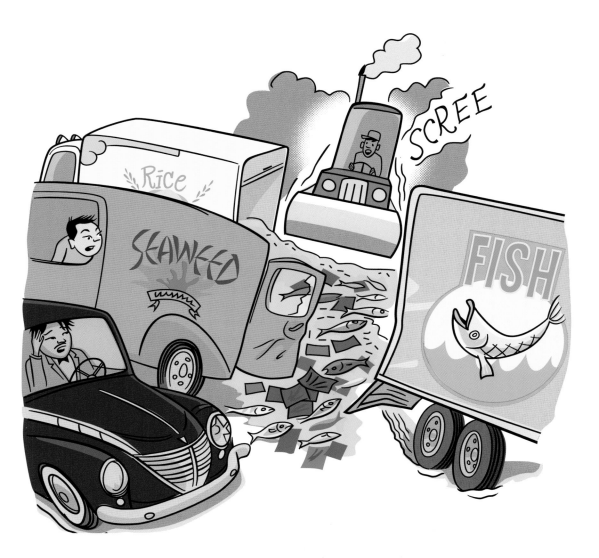

Grocery Store Coupons

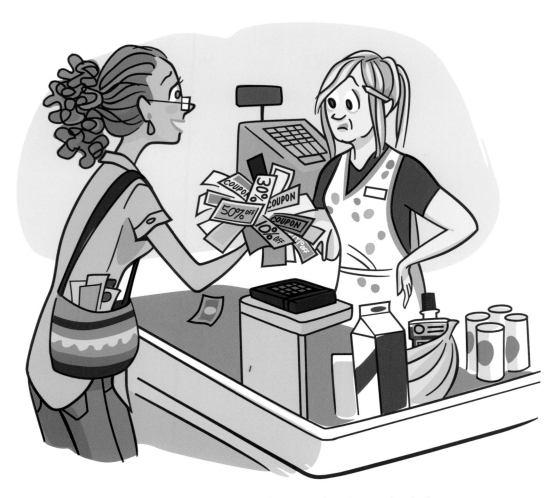

"It appears you owe me $400 and a chopped salad!"

American Idle

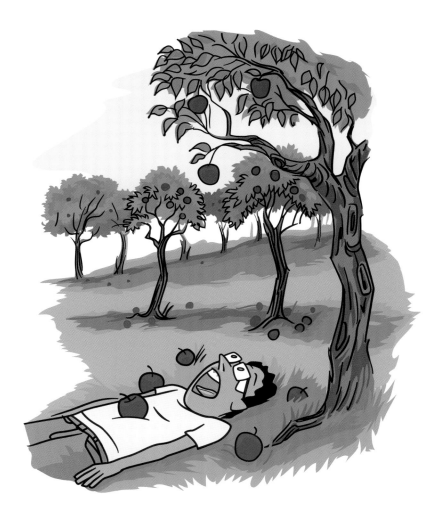

Gerald had discovered a whole new kind of lazy.

Half a Laugh

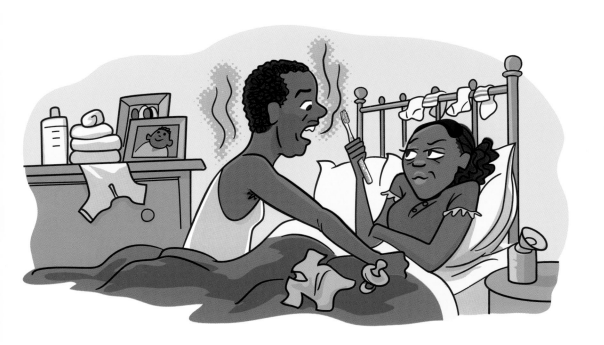

(Insert your caption here.)

Dear Reader,

We believe that laughter is truly the best medicine. That's why we co-developed this book inspired by funny moments in everyday life to help everyone achieve their healthiest, happiest smiles.

One of our favorite illustrations (Bedtime Performance Art) reveals the absurdity of our evening rituals and the humor of what we go through to look and feel our best. While this scene gives us a chuckle, it also reminds us that we need to do our part to achieve a healthy smile by brushing, flossing, and rinsing every day.

To ensure America's children spend more time on the playground and less time in the dentist's chair, we have made a donation to the National Children's Oral Health Foundation®: America's Toothfairy for each book produced. We encourage you to keep the laughter coming by visiting www.AmericasToothfairy.org and helping to give back.

Regards,

The makers of LISTERINE® TOTAL CARE and REACH® TOTAL CARE products